Intermittent Fasting

The Ultimate Natural Weight Loss, Rejuvenation, And Anti-aging Guide

(Utilize The Well-known Intermittent Fasting Diet Plan To Maintain Your Health)

Marshall Campbell

TABLE OF CONTENT

chapter 1: What Are The Benefits Of Intermittent Fasting? Which Is It? 1

Chapter 2: The Advantages And Detriments Of Intermittent Fasting 5

Chapter 4: Popular Diet Programs 19

Chapter 5: Beginning If Critical Success Factors 22

Chapter 8: How Should One Start A Fasting Regimen? 28

Chapter 9: Starting Intermittent Fasting 32

Chapter 10: Among The Prevalent Fasting Patterns Are 35

Chapter 11: Plan Meals According To Your Easy Eating Window 38

Chapter 13: How To Safely Exercise During Intermittent Fasting 46

Chapter 14: The Changes Women Over 50 Are Bound To Face And How To Approach This Nutritionally 49

Chapter 16: Your Hormones And Your Cells. 58

Chapter 17: Methods Involving Intermittent Fasting 63

Chapter 18: Benefits Of Intermittent Fasting For Older Women 65

Chapter 19: Effect Of Intermittent Fasting 72

Chapter 1: What Are The Benefits Of Intermittent Fasting? Which Is It?

Your body can only exist in one of two states: fed or fasted. In fact, you are currently in one of these states! Since we have been brainwashed into believing that the more meals we easy eat, the faster our metabolisms will function, even if you are an average American who easy eats breakfast, lunch, dinner, and snacks in between, you wake up every morning in a fasting state. Breakfast is the first meal of the day because it breaks the fasting period of the previous night. Therefore, felicitations! You are already fasting EVERY SINGLE DAY OF YOUR LIFE. When framed in this manner, fasting doesn't sound quite so peculiar, does it?

You were unaware that you were already moving faster!

The only thing left to do now that we know you ALREADY fast every single day is to lengthen the fast   Since you do not wake up during the night to easy eat, we can assume that your body is already capable of fasting.

HOWEVER, WHY SHOULD WE FAST? It appears to be the best part. Fasting has a metabolic advantage over other easily weight loss strategies. Basically Remember from the "calories" chapter that our metabolisms slow down to protect us when they detect a caloric deficit. The Biggest Loser study made us aware of this fact. The key to any easily weight loss strategy being really effective is preventing our bodies from detecting a calorie deficit. Therein lies the power of fasting. You really become a fat-burning machine during the fast when your body adapts to fasting. You may need the energy stored in your fat reserves to get through the day. That is, after all, why it is stored there. Here's how the magic works: because you have PLENTY of stored energy on your body AND can now access it efficiently, your body does not perceive an energy deficit. This is ENORMOUS NEWS, people! Unlike the metabolisms of the contestants on The Biggest Loser, your metabolism does not slow down.

In addition to increasing resting energy expenditure, intermittent fasting has a number of health benefits that are currently being studied by the medical research community.

Simple discuss autophagy. It is a natural process taking place within your body. This is how your body eliminates excess "trash" cells. To simplify, think of it as your body's own recycling system, which is how your cells eliminate waste. Why is autophagy essential for survival? A buildup of excessive cellular "debris" is the root cause of a variety of age-related diseases and conditions. If you don't give your body a chance to eliminate waste, your entire system will really become clogged. Think about how your family may react to this. If you stopped taking the garbage out, chaos would quickly ensue. Autophagy is necessary for the maintenance of a healthy body. the previously mentioned website link Parkinson's disease, type 2 diabetes, and other geriatric disorders have all been linked to autophagy disruption. Mutations in autophagy-related genes can result in inherited disease. There is a correlation between cancer and autophagic system dysfunction.

Chapter 2: The Advantages And Detriments Of Intermittent Fasting

Intermittent fasting (IF) has been used to easy eat a variety of ailments for millennia.

There are numerous same different types of intermittent fasting, ranging from plans that prohibit meals on specific days to protocols that restrict easy eating only at specific times.

Even healthy individuals can adopt these easy eating habits to easily achieve and maintain a healthy weight and reap the benefits of wellness.

The benefits and drawbacks of intermittent fasting are still under investigation. Long-term research is required to determine whether this diet has lasting benefits.

Gewicht loss

Research suggests that intermittent fasting can aid in easily weight loss and control.

By lowering insulin levels, intermittent fasting may facilitate weight loss.

The body breaks down carbohydrates into glucose, which cells use for energy or convert into fat for later use. Insulin is a hormone that facilitates glucose absorption by cells.

In the absence of food, insulin levels decline. It is likely that during a fast, decreased insulin levels cause cells to release their glucose reserves as a source of energy.

Regarding weight loss, both diet types were equally effective.

Other health indicators, simply including blood pressure and heart rate, did not differ significantly between the groups.

The majority of recent studies indicate that intermittent fasting may be an really effective method for weight loss.

Although it is unlikely to be more really effective than conventional calorie restriction, some individuals may find intermittent fasting to be more convenient.

A lower risk of developing type 2 diabetes
Intermittent fasting may also be advantageous for diabetes prevention because it can aid in easily weight loss and may really affect other characteristics associated with an increased risk of diabetes.

A major risk factor for developing type 2 diabetes is being overweight or obese.

However, additional research is necessary to determine if intermittent fasting can prevent type 2 diabetes.

Researchers discovered decreases in diabetes indicators such as insulin sensitivity in overweight and obese individuals.

In light of this, they believe that intermittent fasting may easy reduce the prevalence of type 2 diabetes in this population.

Nevertheless, according to rat research published in the journal Endocrine Abstracts in 2018, intermittent fasting may easily increase the risk of developing diabetes.

Over the course of three months, researchers tracked the effects of intermittent fasting in rats.

While weight and food intake were reduced, there was an easily increase in abdominal fat tissue, a decrease in muscle, and signs that the body was not processing insulin correctly. These are diabetes type 2 risk factors.

The results of this study must be replicated, and additional research is required to determine whether these findings in rats are applicable to humans.

Enhances cognitive
According to animal studies, intermittent fasting improves cognitive function.

Intermittent fasting may enhance brain health by decreasing inflammation.

According to one study, mice on a brief intermittent fasting diet demonstrated superior learning and memory compared to mice with unrestricted access to food.

Further animal research indicates that intermittent fasting can easy reduce inflammation in the brain, which has been associated with neurological disorders.

Other animal research has discovered that intermittent fasting can easy reduce the risk of neurological diseases such as Alzheimer's, Parkinson's, and stroke.

The applicability of these findings to humans requires additional research.

Chapter 3: Simply avoid These Mistakes During Intermittent Fasting

Intermittent fasting is a technique that is gaining popularity today. When one has tried everything to lose weight without success, it is difficult not to be tempted by the latter because it is so really effective and simple to implement. Briefly, intermittent fasting is the practice of alternating periods of fasting with healthy **easy eat**ing. Here is a list of mistakes to simply avoid during the first weeks of fasting so as not to be disappointed.

EXPECT A MIRACLE
Some people may complain about not losing more than 5 kg in a month of intermittent fasting, which is ludicrous because there are so many others who would be thrilled to lose half that

amount by **easy eat**ing whatever they really want and not exercising. Intermittent fasting is beneficial for weight loss, but you should not dream. You must allow your body sufficient time to shed those extra pounds at its own pace.

EASY EAT ANYTHING

I practice intermittent fasting because I enjoy being able to consume all of my favorite foods. As a result, it is very easy to consume one or two burgers and a large portion of fries liberally covered in mayonnaise and ketchup. If you consume an excessive amount of high-calorie foods, you will not be able to lose weight through intermittent fasting.

DO NOT MOVE ENOUGH

You wait until the weekend to fast because you are calm on the weekend.

The concern is that after a few hours of inactivity, you will begin to feel hungry and your mind will wander. Indeed, it is impossible not to consider snack packs when spending the day on the couch watching television. You do not need to move less if you do not consume food. You have sufficient energy reserves to live normally and move freely. Take advantage of your fasting day by walking, working, tinkering, etc. Being busy will distract you from your desire to snack.

DO NOT DRINK ENOUGH WATER

You believe your body is requesting food when, in reality, you are simply dehydrated. During the fasting period, it is essential to consume a lot of water.

DRINK EXCESSIVE COFFEE

What is more tempting than allegedly fooling the hungry by squatting the coffee maker? In fact, those who practice intermittent fasting typically substitute coffee without sugar for breakfast. This is perfectly normal given that caffeine provides a tonic, aids in combating hunger, and can boost the metabolism. That does not imply that you must consume a liter of water.

TO BE A LITTLE TOO OPTIMISTIC

If you are convinced of the advantages of intermittent fasting, you may be tempted to begin with a 24-hour fast. Error! This is the best way to demotivate you, as your first failure will disgust you. To acclimate your body to this new lifestyle, you should begin gradually but consistently. Start, for instance, by delaying or skipping breakfast and **easy eat**ing lunch earlier. After that, you will gradually quicken your pace. You will quickly adjust to the new circumstances.

DO A LITTLE TOO MUCH

Motivated by the outcome, you set the bar higher, or even too high, by fasting for two consecutive days. Again, you commit a grave error, as I am referring to intermittent fasting, which is periodic but not permanent. After twenty-four hours, the benefits of this method begin to diminish. Therefore, it serves no purpose to starve yourself further. Your body may react negatively otherwise, and you will experience the opposite effect.

Make a determination regarding the schedules.
When just beginning intermittent fasting, it is somewhat normal to have your eyes glued to the clock. However,

this reflex must gradually disappear. It is completely pointless and even counterproductive to begin counting down at 10:00 a.m. if your first meal is not scheduled until 4:00 p.m.

BEING TOO HARD ON YOURSELF

Discipline is a virtue. However, do not overdo it. You can break the fast 30 minutes to an hour beforehand without compromising your efforts. Under the guise that it is not yet time, it is unnecessary to inflict long minutes of torture. In addition, the large amount of cortisol produced by stress will cause more really damage than the cheese that softens the eyes.

The same applies to what must or must not be consumed during the fasting period. During fasting, you can drink water, coffee, and tea without sugar, as well as non-caloric supplements such as vitamins and minerals. But if you are too tired and hungry during the day, you can add a small spoonful of cream to your coffee without just feeling guilty. There are no strict rules; everything is balanced. Basically Remember that you must adhere to the outline, but that does not mean you must take charge of the details. Learn to live your new lifestyle with composure.

ABUSE "LIGHT" DRINKS

A zero Coke technically contains zero calories. So, you may reason, why not chain the cans to decorate the fasting day? However, you should be aware that artificial sweeteners stimulate insulin secretion. As a result, they inhibit your production of growth hormone. With intermittent fasting, you really want to simply avoid precisely this effect. To maximize your performance, simply avoid this beverage. However, if you are content with a moderate amount and that it is an occasional occurrence, why not?

Chapter 4: Popular Diet Programs

In the previous chapter, I discussed the significance of a balanced diet and how it contributes to the efficacy of intermittent fasting. However, I am aware that many individuals who are successfully adhering to particular diet plans, especially if they are attempting to reach a specific easily weight loss goal, will also wish to continue their diet.

Certainly, you can combine intermittent fasting with a diet that works for you.

It is essential to realize that both dieting and fasting can have a significant effect on your metabolism. It will require some adjusting. However, one that is well worthwhile.

Let me also mention that, regardless of the diet you choose, it is essential to continue consuming the minimum daily requirements for all nutrients.

If this describes you, you may benefit from intermittent fasting. Therefore, allow me to briefly simple discuss popular diets and IF.

High-Protein Diet

In Chapter 11, I stated that 10%–35% of your daily calories should come from protein, depending on your level of activity. Within this range, a high-protein diet begins with 20% of your daily calories coming from protein. Additionally, these diets limit carbohydrates and sometimes vegetables. Atkins and the Zone are two well-known high-protein diets.

High-protein diets are really effective for easily weight loss because when you consume fewer carbohydrates, your body runs out of blood sugar during fasting more quickly.

In an earlier chapter, I discussed some of the risks of consuming an excessive amount of protein. In addition, you may gain weight because many protein sources are high in calories. Others find that a high-protein diet causes gastrointestinal issues.

Chapter 5: Beginning If Critical Success Factors

After completing this, I also explain why they need these things and how their thought process will be same different if they easily achieve these objectives. This will teach you what matters to you. Despite the fact that external factors frequently really affect our objectives, they must ultimately be relevant to you. Develop a strategy for your data analysis:

Organization

Perform a schedule audit! Many individuals choose a mealtime only to discover that they will need more time to easy eat there. Not a good beginning! Consider where you may have difficulty surviving without food. For instance, if you easy eat when bored, setting your fasting window during the slowest part of your day is not a good idea. Consider your family dining habits when determining your easy eating window. Select your feeding window with care. Make the procedure as straightforward as possible for yourself.

It is essential to have positive people in your life who are also on the same path. It will really become difficult, and you will need to stop periodically. Support from others is essential to success and can mean the same difference between easily giving up and persisting!

Chapter 6: Additional Potential Advantages of Intermittent Fasting

Simple to implement. Because technically no foods are restricted, intermittent fasting is easier to adhere to than conventional dieting, which is one of its greatest advantages.

Simple meal preparation. Since less food must be prepared and cleaned up, meal planning is simplified and made easier, making it ideal for busy people.

- Enhanced metabolic rate According to a number of studies, intermittent fasting preserves lean muscle mass more effectively than calorie-restricted diets while affecting the metabolism less negatively than calorie-restricted diets.

- Possible financial savings. By easy eating at home more often and purchasing fewer groceries, you can easy reduce your expenses.

- Mental tranquility It is an excellent alternative for those who do not wish to monitor their food intake and count calories.

- Improve the brain's health. Animal studies suggest that fasting may improve memory and cognitive function. Furthermore, it may easy reduce the risk of neurodegenerative diseases such as Parkinson's and Alzheimer's. More research is needed to determine whether these benefits also apply to humans.

Chapter 7: How long does it take to see results after initiating an intermittent fast?

The rate at which extra weight begins to diminish depends on a variety of factors. The rate of easily weight loss will vary significantly from person to person based on a number of factors, simply including initial weight, intermittent fasting method, "easy eating windows," and others.

Rapid easily weight loss is possible if you immediately begin calorie restriction and maintain a healthy calorie deficit (consuming fewer calories than you burn). Any initial easily weight loss is "likely to be water weight," and real results will not be visible for at least two weeks.

It is possible to lose between one and two pounds per week through intermittent fasting, depending on the number of calories consumed. This may necessitate a wait of eight to ten weeks before you notice any progress.

What exactly are you forfeiting if your losses exceed that threshold? This could be a warning sign. If you begin an intermittent fasting plan and lose a significant amount of weight rapidly, you should reevaluate your calorie intake to ensure you're still meeting your body's needs.

Chapter 8: How Should One Start A Fasting Regimen?

Although you may not have recognized it yet, the concept of intermittent fasting has already appeared frequently in our lives. Regardless of how frequently or infrequently we skip meals, skipping breakfast or lunch can be considered a form of intermittent fasting. Regardless of how frequently or infrequently we skip meals, this is true. Intermittent fasting can aid in weight loss.

You must start by selecting one of the above-mentioned strategies, determining which one is most suitable for your lifestyle and available time, and then putting that method to the test. Do not have a rocky beginning. If you don't take things slowly when utilizing the

16:8 method, you may find yourself wanting to quit after only a few days.

Getting Started

There is a good chance that you have participated in multiple intermittent fasts over the course of your lifetime.

If you have ever easy eaten dinner, gone to bed late, and then skipped breakfast, lunch, and dinner the following day, you have likely experienced a fast lasting longer than 16 hours.

Constantly, some individuals consume food in this manner. Simply put, they do not experience morning feelings of hunger.

It is recommended that you begin intermittent fasting with the 16:8 technique, as many consider it to be the simplest and most manageable method.

If you find that fasting is not difficult and you feel good while doing so, you should consider more advanced fasts such as 24-hour fasts one to two times per week (Easy eat-Stop-Easy eat) or consuming 500 to 600 calories one to two days per week (5:2 diet).

Another method is to simply abstain from food whenever possible; for instance, you could skip meals when you are not hungry or when you do not have time to prepare food.

It is not necessary to adhere to a specific intermittent fasting strategy in order to reap at least some of the benefits of intermittent fasting.

Experiment with the various techniques and find something that fits your schedule and that you enjoy doing.

Chapter 9: Starting Intermittent Fasting

How long does it take to see easily weight loss results? There is no definitive timeline for the results of intermittent fasting. However, based on scientific evidence and reported personal experience, there is an average amount of time to anticipate easily weight loss that is measurable. With this method of intermittent fasting, there are no daily calorie or time restrictions, and you can easy eat whatever you want—but only 500 calories the following day.

Due to differences in metabolism, amount of physical activity, dietary choices, sleep schedules, stress levels, and exposure to toxins, these outcomes vary from person to person. If easily weight loss is your top priority, you should fast for longer. The longer you fast, the more fat you will burn and the more really effective your results will be. A weight scale is merely a tool for measuring progress, and its accuracy is not always optimal. Scales provide instantaneous measurements, and his weight varies throughout the day. Consistently weigh yourself each day at the same time if you wish to monitor your progress. Initially in the morning is optimal.

Why you should not depend on the scale. Along with the scale, grab a tape measure and measure your torso, hips, abdomen, and lower body every month in centimeters. During intermittent fasting, the body alters its shape by storing fat and primarily maintaining or gaining muscle mass (this also depends on your physical activity).

Because of this, the success of intermittent fasting is frequently measured in terms of inches lost rather than significant weight loss. One report

In six months, a woman's visceral fat increased by four percentage points. 2% To 7%. After one week of intermittent fasting, you will experience less abdominal bloating and a more toned, firmer core. Some people experience easily weight loss during the second week, but don't be disheartened if you don't. Continue for an additional 4 to 6 weeks, and you should observe changes. Expect to lose a pound or two per week and a few inches per month if you gain weight.

Chapter 10: Among The Prevalent Fasting Patterns Are

This consists of a 16-hour fast followed by an 8-hour easy eating window. It's one of the simplest forms of fasting, and you've likely practiced it without realizing it. For example, if you ate dinner at 7 p.m. and breakfast at 7 a.m., you've already fasted for 12 hours. This fasting method is adaptable to your needs.

You can switch to a 9 a.m. to 5 p.m. easy eating window, 7 a.m. to 3 p.m., etc. Water, 1 tsp of lemon/apple cider vinegar in water, coffee, and herbal tea can provide relief during fasting periods. The effectiveness of intermittent fasting typically occurs during the night and early morning, which is why it is sometimes beneficial to extend breakfast until noon.

The 5:2 diet is a type of fast in which a person easy eats normally for 5 days, followed by 2 days of fasting and easy eating meals of no more than 500/600 calories.

One meal a day (OMAD) fasting consists of easy eating one meal per day and fasting for the remainder of the day.

Alternate Day: As the name suggests, alternate day fasting involves easy eating normally one day and then fasting the next.

Chapter 11: Plan Meals According To Your Easy Eating Window

After choosing an intermittent fasting method, the next step is to plan your meals accordingly. This involves choosing foods that will keep you full and satisfied during your easy eating window and adhering to this schedule for optimal results.

Prepare and plan your meals
To successfully implement intermittent fasting, it is essential to plan and prepare your meals in advance. This will ensure that you continue to meet your nutritional requirements during the designated easy eating periods. This will ensure that you continue to meet your nutritional needs during mealtime.

In addition to planning your meals, it is essential to stay hydrated and consume sufficient nutrients from whole, unprocessed foods.

Include nutrient-dense foods like leafy greens, lean protein, healthy fats, and fiber in your diets.

Experiment with various recipes to discover tasty and filling meals.

After selecting a method of intermittent fasting, the next step is to begin gradually. This involves gradually incorporating fasting into your daily routine and paying attention to your body's requirements. It is essential to simply avoid excessive exercise or dietary restriction in the beginning, as it can result in fatigue, dizziness, or nausea.

Start by abstaining from food for 12 to 16 hours per day and work your way up to 24 hours. You may find it beneficial to start by fasting every other day or by dividing your fasting days between the weekdays and weekends. Basically Remember to drink plenty of fluids (non-caloric beverages) and to break your fast gradually with a light meal.

While intermittent fasting can result in weight loss, it is essential to also engage in regular physical activity. This may include cardiovascular exercises such as walking or running, in addition to strength training with weights or resistance bands. Aim for at least 30 minutes of daily exercise and pay attention to your body's requirements.

Chapter 12: Dietary Strategies That Complement Intermittent Fasting

Intermittent fasting is not a diet, but it has proven to be an really effective method of weight loss. However, if you do not adhere to a healthy diet while on this fast, you may experience negative effects. For instance, if after breaking the fast you consume a large amount of junk food and sweets, you may gain weight.

Similarly, if you consume a 3,000-calorie meal simply because you are fasting, you may not experience the benefits of the fast. This has prompted discussions about the optimal diet to pair with intermittent fasting.

This article will examine diets that have been demonstrated to be compatible with intermittent fasting.

The keto diet, also known as the ketogenic diet, is a high-fat, low-carbohydrate diet that induces a state that makes it easier for the body to burn fat. This condition is known as ketosis. Ketosis occurs when the body is unable to use glucose for energy and instead burns fat for fuel.

When the body begins to burn fat for energy, it has entered the state of ketosis. The ketogenic diet has existed for a very long time, but it has never been used for weight loss. In the past, it was more commonly used to treasy eat health problems such as epilepsy. Ketosis is known to have a beneficial effect on the brain, reducing seizures as a result.

This diet also protects the brain from Alzheimer's disease and inflammation. It has also been shown to easy reduce blood glucose levels in Type II diabetics. However, the diet has recently gained popularity due to its easily weight loss effects.

This diet requires you to consume very few carbohydrates, typically less than 25 grams per day, minimal protein, and an abundance of fat. Ideal meal composition would consist of 5% carbohydrates, 20% protein, and 75% fat.

Although this diet permits a high fat intake, healthy fats such as avocado, cheese, cream, and grass-fed butter are encouraged. This diet discourages sugary foods and alcohol consumption.

The time required to enter ketosis varies among individuals.

Combining intermittent fasting and the ketogenic diet can augment the effects of each in a number of ways. They are discussed further below.

1. Reach Ketosis Sooner

Fasting reduces carbohydrate consumption, and if this continues for an extended period of time, the body will run out of glucose. This forces the body to use fat as fuel. Therefore, your body will enter ketosis faster.

The combination of a diet and fast can easily increase fat burning.

Since fasting can facilitate rapid ketosis, many individuals group their keto meals. Consequently, they include meals in their fasting schedule. Since calories are not accumulated throughout the day, fat will be burned.

3. The state of ketosis reduces hunger

The hunger hormone (ghrelin) is suppressed during ketosis. Therefore, you can fast for a longer period of time without just feeling hungry.

Intermittent fasting promotes muscle growth

Intermittent fasting stimulates growth hormone, which aids in muscle growth. This is beneficial because keto does not promote muscle growth.

Chapter 13: How To Safely Exercise During Intermittent Fasting

The success of any easily weight loss or exercise program is contingent upon its ability to be maintained over time. If your ultimate goal is to easy reduce body fat and maintain your fitness level while using intermittent fasting, you must remain in the safe zone. Here are some specific tips to assist you in doing so.

Consume a meal prior to your moderate- to vigorous-intensity workout.

This is the point where meal timing enters rlau. Timing a meal prior to a moderate- or high-intensity workout is advisable, according to Khorana au. Thus, your body will have access to glucose stores to fuel your workout.

Stau hudrated

Sonral au to basically Remember fating does not imply water removal. He suggests that you consume more water while fasting.

According to Sonpal, a good source of hydration that is low in calories is coconut water. He states, "It replenishes electrolytes, is low in calories, and tastes pretty good." Gatorade and rort drinks are high in sugar, so limit your consumption.

Maintain moderate intensity and duration

If you overexert yourself and begin to feel dizzy or faint, take a break. Listening to one's body is essential.

Consider the fat type.

If you are following a 24-hour intermittent fast, you should stick to low-intensity exercises such as walking, restorative yoga, and gentle pilates. But if you're doing the 16:8 fast, the majority of the 16-hour fasting window occurs in the evening, at night, and early in the morning, so committing to a specific exercise regimen is not essential.

Observe your body

The most important piece of advice to follow when exercising during IF is to pay attention to your body. "If you begin to feel weak or dizzy, chances are you have low blood sugar or are dehydrated," Amengual explained. If this is the case, he should consume an electrolyte-sugar drink immediately, followed by a well-balanced meal.

While intermittent fasting and exercise may be really effective for some roles, others may not feel comfortable engaging in any form of exercise while fasting. Consult your physician or healthcare provider before beginning any diet or exercise regimen.

Chapter 14: The Changes Women Over 50 Are Bound To Face And How To Approach This Nutritionally

Mood and Sleeplessness during Menopause

It is common for women to experience irritability during this time in their lives. This can negatively impact the decision-making process regarding our health care. Additionally, insomnia can worsen this stage. Although neither situation has a solution, both can be approached from a nutritional standpoint. How? Consuming foods that promote emotional health, relaxation, and serotonin synthesis. For instance, dark chocolate, cinnamon-spiked hot milk, bananas, and nuts.

Deficient Energy

Additionally, fatigue is prevalent at this stage. Therefore, it is essential to adhere to a well-planned diet consisting of small but regular meals. For example, five to seven meals. Also, simply avoid foods that can exacerbate feelings of fatigue, such as refined sugars and caffeinated beverages. Sugars produce an on-off effect that results in a subsequent drop in blood sugar levels. Caffeine- and caffeine-containing beverages, such as coffee and tea, should not be avoided, but their consumption should be regulated because they impair sleep and cause fatigue and lack of energy.

Bone Decalcification Upon Disappearance of Menstruation

The protective effect of estrogens on bone tissue. When a woman's body stops producing them, changes in calcium regulation occur, resulting in a loss of bone mass. On a nutritional level, we must prevent bone loss through three primary factors:

Milk, yogurt, almonds, orange, broccoli, and cabbage provide calcium.

Taking in less salt facilitates the excretion of calcium through urine.

Ensuring a sufficient supply of exogenous vitamin D (through food and/or supplements) and endogenous vitamin D (the body itself manufactured with sun exposure).

In addition to minimizing the consumption of decalcifying substances such as sugar and carbonated beverages.

Cardiovascular Risk

The risk of cardiovascular disease increases after menopause. Typically, cholesterol levels tend to rise. We suggest adopting a heart-healthy diet by consuming more healthy fats (extra virgin olive oil, nuts, and avocado) and avoiding saturated and Trans fats (cheeses, sausages) (processed foods such as chips, cereal bars, and cookies).

Body Fat Redistribution and Weight Gain

Physically speaking, the most noticeable and annoying aspect of menopause is weight gain. At this stage of life, fat no longer accumulates predominantly in the hips, but rather in the belly or abdomen. In addition to increasing cardiovascular risk, cholesterol, and blood pressure, this factor also increases the likelihood of cardiovascular disease. This indicates that we will likely have to watch what we easy eat more closely and possibly adopt a low-calorie diet.

Lower Muscle Mass

Inadequate weight gain is accompanied by a reduction in muscle mass. This change is inevitable, but we must prepare for it by consuming a diet rich in lean proteins (rabbit, turkey, and white fish) and engaging in strength or toning exercises.

Finally, it is important to highlight some common dietary changes that occur in women during menopause due to new food preferences or attempts to lose weight. This is typically reflected in dinners, which consist of yogurt, salad, or bread. This can exacerbate weight gain and muscle mass loss caused by a lack of protein and cooked vegetables.

Menopause hormone fluctuations can cause fluid retention. This factor does not really affect every woman in the same way. Similarly to how some women retain fluids during menstruation and others do not, the same occurs at this stage. Changes in estrogen levels influence the water balance of the body. How can fluid retention be treasy eated? Consuming less salt, increasing fiber- and antioxidant-rich vegetables, consuming copious amounts of water, and engaging in regular physical activity are all recommended.

Easy reduce fluid retention during menopause by consuming less salt, fiber-rich vegetables, and antioxidants. Do not forget to exercise and drink plenty of water.

Chapter 15: Has Intermittent Fasting (IF) any side effects?

Even though intermittent fasting has medical benefits that everyone can appreciate, this does not imply that everyone can benefit from it. Fasting strategies, like any other weight-loss technique, are not reasonable or attainable for all individuals.

Hunger, Weakness, Slow Responses, Cravings, and Dehydration are a few of the mild secondary effects that can be triggered by fasting.

It is normal for any of these side effects to occur. However, if they persist and do not subside after a short time, you should discontinue your chosen fasting method and consult your primary care doctor. There may be fundamental medical issues. Fasting is not appropriate for all individuals. It depends on the individual's ongoing lifestyle and health conditions. Anyone with basic medical issues or concerns should abstain from fasting and not begin before consulting a medical professional. There are a variety of health risks associated with irregular fasting:

Patients diabetic

Anyone with current or historical dietary problems

Low systolic pulse

Persons with a low BMI

Women attempting to conceive Women with current or previous amenorrhea

Expectant or nursing mothers

If you wish to try fasting but have any of the aforementioned concerns, you should consult a professional beforehand. Fasting can have significant negative effects on your health and occasionally worsen your ongoing condition.

Chapter 16: Your Hormones And Your Cells

During fasting, your body undergoes numerous cellular and molecular changes, such as modifying hormone levels to easily increase the availability of stored body fat.

In addition, your cells initiate vital repair processes and alter gene expression, and while intermittent fasting may aid in weight loss, it may also really affect hormone levels. This is because the body stores energy in body fat (calories), and when you don't easy eat, your body does several things to make the stored energy more usable.

Examples include the activity of the nervous system and the levels of numerous important hormones. During a fast, the body undergoes the following modifications:

Human Growth Hormone (HGH) Levels: soaring by a factor of five at times. This has benefits for, among other things, muscle growth and fat loss.

Insulin: Insulin sensitivity improves and insulin levels drop precipitously. Reduced insulin levels enhance the utilization of fat reserves.

Self-repair of cells: When you fast, your cells begin repairing themselves. This includes autophagy, in which cells degrade and eliminate accumulated damaged and obsolete proteins.

The operation of the genes involved in aging and disease prevention undergoes alterations.

Epinephrine (noradrenaline) (noradrenaline). The nervous system sends the neurotransmitter norepinephrine to fat cells, causing them to convert body fat into free fatty acids that can be used as fuel.

Contrary to what some proponents of five- to six-times-a-day easy eating suggest, short-term fasting may easily increase fat-burning. According to research, trials of whole-day fasting lasting 12–24 weeks and trials of alternate-day fasting lasting 3–12 weeks both aid in easily weight loss and fat loss.

Human growth hormone (HGH), whose levels can easily increase up to fivefold during a fast, is another hormone whose levels change. Previously, it was believed that HGH accelerated fat burning, but a recent study indicates that hormones may signal the brain to conserve energy, making easily weight loss more difficult.

By stimulating a limited number of agouti-related protein (AgRP) neurons, HGH may indirectly easily increase hunger and slow down energy metabolism.

SUMMARY

A brief fast induces a number of physiological modifications that promote fat burning. However, elevated HGH levels can indirectly inhibit energy metabolism and impede weight loss. The health benefits of intermittent fasting stem from alterations in hormone levels, cell structure, and gene expression.

During fasting, insulin levels fall and human growth hormone levels rise. In addition, your cells modify gene expression and initiate vital cellular repair processes.

Chapter 17: Methods Involving Intermittent Fasting

Understanding how to intermittently fast is essential for maintaining a balanced diet and avoiding unnecessary risks. There is never a single really effective easily weight loss strategy. Some individuals may be able to sustain intermittent fasting, whereas others may find that this method is not suitable for them.

If you really want to try intermittent fasting, you must first determine how this easy eating pattern will fit into your lifestyle, especially in terms of social gatherings and physical activity.

There are many same different types of intermittent fasting plans. Before beginning an intermittent fasting regimen, you must consult your physician. Once you have obtained their approval, the actual procedure is simple.

To be successful with intermittent fasting, you must determine the plan that best suits you. It must be compatible with your regular schedules, exercise regimens, and social obligations.

Because there are so many varieties, it can be challenging to know where to begin. Some are more difficult than others, requiring longer periods of fasting, whereas faster methods may not be really effective for your objectives.

Chapter 18: Benefits Of Intermittent Fasting For Older Women

Intermittent fasting has additional advantages beyond weight loss. Fasting has been a tradition since the beginning of time, and it is still regularly observed in many cultures today. For women over 50, attempting to lose weight can be extremely difficult. This could be due to a number of factors, the majority of which are adverse effects of diet culture and fad diets. In terms of fitness, nutrition, and weight loss, women over the age of 50 feel extremely lost today. It promotes the notion that restriction and deprivation are necessary for easily weight loss and maintenance.

Constraint and deprivation cannot be sustained. Everything that is not sustainable is a waste of time, money, and resources. Over the years, I've worked with a large number of women over the age of 50, and many of them have tried virtually every diet imaginable to the point of easily giving up.

Other physiological issues can manifest in women over 50.

Menopause can cause hormonal changes and a decrease in lean body mass (muscle), both of which can slow the metabolism.

This could imply that once-beneficial methods for women over 50 are no longer as effective. Intermittent fasting can be an really effective method for women over 50 to easy reduce stubborn body fat, manage hunger, and easily increase energy.

Medical metabolite

Some women can experience the onset of menopause in their fifties. A woman's body undergoes observable changes during menopause, simply including a slowing of the metabolism, a loss of muscle mass, and hormonal shifts. Women over the age of 50 who engage in intermittent fasting may experience improvements in blood pressure, visceral fat, and insulin sensitivity. Fasting can also be used to manage and monitor the aging of your metabolism.

elevated levels of energy

Without constant digestion, you have more energy for other activities. Many women over 50 who transition to intermittent fasting report having constant energy throughout the day. It can seem too liberating to no longer experience energy peaks and valleys.

Improving insulin sensitivity

It has been shown that intermittent fasting increases insulin sensitivity and stabilizes blood sugar levels. I've observed type 2 diabetics regress with this nutritional strategy. Insulin resistance is common in adults over the age of 50, both men and women, but it is not an inevitable consequence of aging.

Intermittent fasting boosts ketone levels

During a fast, the body depletes its supply of glucose, which is typically restored by consuming carbohydrates and proteins. Although glucose is the body's preferred energy source, fasting forces the body to switch to another source.

By metabolizing fat in the liver in the absence of glucose, the body produces ketones, a readily usable form of energy. Ketones provide energy for the muscles, heart, and brain, which are absorbed by the mitochondria.

Certain parts of the body, notably the brain, cannot utilize ketones and must instead rely on glucose. This glucose is produced through gluconeogenesis, a process that also involves the breakdown of lipid glycerol and proteins. Alzheimer's disease may serve as a prime example of the potential anti-aging effects of ketones.

Alzheimer's disease and glucose metabolism are linked. This is the rationale behind Alzheimer's disease being classified as type 3 diabetes. By avoiding the negative effects of suboptimal glucose metabolism, ketones can directly provide energy to the brain and enhance cognitive performance in Alzheimer's disease patients.

Ketosis induced by dietary modifications can improve memory in elderly individuals with cognitive impairment. Ketosis, which is induced by intermittent fasting, would therefore be expected to slow the aging of the brain.

There is evidence that regular intermittent fasting makes cells more resistant to oxidative responses. This cellular resilience is the result of hormesis, the process of defining advantageous biological responses to stress.

Exercising and easy eating healthy foods are two examples of hormesis. Both exercise and specific phytochemicals found in vegetables can cause the body to experience some stress. However, exercise and vegetables are advantageous because the body handles stress well.

Intermittent fasting is an additional illustration of hormesis. Excessive fasting would result in the breakdown of muscle tissue and deasy eath. However, a small amount of stress from fasting every day is sufficient to prevent negative effects and initiate beneficial biological processes that, over time, easily increase your resistance to oxidative stress, one of the primary contributors to aging and degenerative diseases.

Chapter 19: Effect Of Intermittent Fasting

Intermittent fasting can be beneficial for weight loss, but it can also really affect your hormones.

Due to the fact that the body stores excess energy as fat, this is the case.

When you go without food for an extended period of time, your body undergoes a series of changes to make the stored energy more accessible.

Examples include changes in the activity of the nervous system and significant changes in the levels of a number of essential hormones.

When you fast, your metabolism undergoes the following two modifications:

Insulin. When you easy eat, your insulin levels rise, and when you go without food for a while, they drop significantly.

Having lower insulin levels facilitates fat burning.

Norepinephrine (noradrenaline) (noradrenaline). Your nervous system delivers to your fat cells the hormone norepinephrine, which stimulates them to release free fatty acids. Afterward, these acids can be burned for energy.

Contrary to the assertions of those who advocate easy eating five to six meals per day, it is intriguing to note that short-term fasting may easily increase fat burning.

According to research, both three- to twelve-week trials of alternate-day and twelve- to twenty-four-week trials of whole-day fasting are really effective at reducing body weight and body fat.

However, additional research is necessary to determine the long-term effects of intermittent fasting and easy eating.

Human growth hormone (HGH), whose levels can easily increase by a factor of five during a fast, is yet another hormone whose levels change due to the diet restriction.

In the past, it was believed that HGH helped the body burn fat more quickly; however, recent studies suggest that it may actually signal the brain to conserve energy, making it more difficult to lose excess weight.

By activating a small population of neurons that are related to agouti-related protein, HGH may indirectly stimulate an easily increase in appetite and a decrease in energy metabolism (AgRP).

SUMMARY

When you fast for a short time, your body undergoes a number of changes that can easily increase your fat burning. Despite this, soaring HGH levels may inadvertently slow energy metabolism and impede further weight loss.

Intermittent fasting offers the benefits of consuming fewer calories and losing excess weight.
Intermittent fasting is really effective for easily weight loss in large part because it makes it easier to consume fewer calories overall.
Skipping meals during the fasting periods is a requirement of all protocols.
You will consume fewer calories unless you find a way to compensate by consuming significantly more food during your normal easy eating times.
A 2014 review found that intermittent fasting can easy reduce body weight by between 3 and 8 percent over a three- to twenty-four-week period.
Depending on the rate of weight loss, intermittent fasting may cause easily

weight loss of approximately 0.55 to 1.65 pounds (0.25–0.75 kg) per week.

In addition, people's waist circumference decreased by between 4 and 7 percent, indicating that they lost abdominal fat.

According to these findings, intermittent fasting may be an really effective easily weight loss strategy.

However, the advantages of intermittent fasting extend far beyond merely fat loss.

In addition, it has numerous beneficial effects on metabolic health, and some research suggests that it may even easy reduce the risk of cardiovascular disease.

Even though calorie counting is typically not required when engaging in intermittent fasting, the majority of easily weight loss is due to a general reduction in calorie consumption.

When the amount of calories consumed by each group was held constant, there was no same difference between intermittent fasting and continuous calorie restriction in the amount of weight lost.

A SUMMARY Intermittent fasting is an really effective method of easily weight loss that does not require calorie monitoring. Numerous studies demonstrate its effectiveness in aiding easily weight loss and reducing abdominal fat.

If you are attempting to lose weight while maintaining your muscle mass, intermittent fasting may be able to assist you.

Dieting frequently results in the loss of both fat and muscle, which is one of the most undesirable side effects.

Intermittent fasting may be advantageous for maintaining muscle mass while simultaneously reducing body fat, according to a number of studies.

A recent study found that people who adhered to intermittent calorie restriction lost roughly the same amount of weight as those who adhered to continuous calorie restriction, but with a much more modest loss of muscle mass.

In studies utilizing calorie restriction, 25% of the weight lost was muscle mass, whereas in studies utilizing intermittent calorie restriction, only 10% of the easily weight loss was muscle mass.

Consider, however, that these studies had a number of limitations, so the results should be interpreted with caution. Recent research has shown that, unlike other types of easy eating plans, intermittent fasting has no effect on lean body mass or muscle mass.

SUMMARY

Although there is some evidence to suggest that, compared to conventional methods of calorie restriction, intermittent fasting may allow you to maintain a greasy eater amount of muscle mass, more recent research does not support this notion.

The practice of intermittent fasting makes easy eating healthily much simpler.

Numerous individuals find the ease of implementation to be one of the most appealing aspects of intermittent fasting. The majority of intermittent fasting plans simply require that you keep track of time. There is no need for calorie counting.

The diet that is most advantageous to your health is the one that you will be able to maintain over time. If practicing intermittent fasting makes it easier for you to maintain a healthy diet, it will undoubtedly improve your long-term health and ability to maintain a healthy weight.

IN SUMMARY The ease with which intermittent fasting can facilitate healthy easy eating is one of its primary advantages. This could make it easier to maintain a healthy diet and lifestyle in the long run.

www.ingramcontent.com/pod-product-compliance
Lightning Source LLC
LaVergne TN
LVHW011737060526
838200LV00051B/3200